FOOT REFLEXOLOGY FOR BEGINNERS

Rediscover Balance and Vitality Through Targeted Foot Techniques

ARTHUR FRANCES

Table of Contents

CHAPTER ONE

INTRODUCTION

The theory behind the therapeutic application of foot reflexology is that different body organs and systems are represented by specific points on the feet. By applying pressure to these points, practitioners hope to promote relaxation, reduce stress, and enhance general health. This holistic approach sees the body as a whole and uses the feet as a map of the body's functions.

The History and Origins of Reflexology

Over thousands of years, several ancient civilizations—each with its own traditions and beliefs—developed reflexology, which is where its origins lie.

Ancient Egypt: Around 2330 B.C., reflexology was first recorded in ancient Egypt. Wall paintings discovered in the tomb of an Egyptian physician depict people receiving foot massages. This suggests that foot therapy is a tried-and-true way to promote health and relaxation. The Egyptians believed that applying pressure to specific foot areas could cure illnesses because of their advanced understanding of the human body and its interdependencies.

The principles of Traditional Chinese Medicine (TCM), which has been practiced in China for over 2,500 years, are closely linked to reflexology. By emphasizing the flow of qi (energy) throughout the body, TCM encourages balance and harmony. Reflexology, which maintains that qi blockages can lead to health issues, supports this theory. The Chinese developed specific techniques for stimulating reflex points on the feet in an attempt to aid in healing and restore equilibrium.

Native American Traditions: Native American cultures also employed reflexology in a variety of ways as part of their holistic healing traditions. Pressure points and foot massage were part of the physical and spiritual healing practices of many tribes. Herbal remedies and rituals were often combined with these practices, which focused on a connection to nature and the spirit world. These ancient techniques paved the way for modern reflexology, which has evolved over time but remains firmly grounded in an understanding of the body's interconnected systems.

The Basis of Reflexology in Science

Despite reflexology's long history, its scientific underpinnings are still being investigated. Nerve endings in the feet are believed to be activated by the exercise, sending signals to the brain and other body parts. This interaction is thought to start a series of actions that can promote relaxation, improve circulation, and lessen pain.

Nerve Endings and Body Systems: The feet are home to thousands of nerve endings, each of which represents a different organ or system. It is believed that pressing on these points stimulates the nervous system, enhancing communication between the brain and body. This stimulation can cause a variety of physiological responses, including enhanced blood flow, reduced muscle tension, and better lymphatic drainage.

Stress Reduction: One of the key benefits of reflexology is its ability to reduce stress. By promoting relaxation, reflexology can lower cortisol levels, a hormone linked to stress. This stress reduction may contribute to better general health because chronic stress is linked to several health issues, including weakened immune systems, digestive issues, and cardiovascular disease. Research suggests that reflexology may be helpful in treating pain. Reflexology has been shown to reduce pain in conditions like migraines, fibromyalgia, and arthritis. One of the mechanisms behind this pain relief could be the body's natural painkillers, endorphins, and nerve signal modulation.

Holistic Benefits: Reflexology is commonly used as a complementary therapy in addition to conventional medical treatments. Many practitioners believe it can boost the effectiveness of these treatments by promoting relaxation and improving the patient's overall well-being. In many healthcare settings, including hospitals and wellness centers, it is commonly used to improve quality of life and encourage recovery.

In conclusion

Foot reflexology is a long-standing practice that combines traditional practices with modern scientific understanding. The idea that the body is interconnected is so widely accepted that it has historical roots in Native American, Chinese, and Egyptian cultures. Even though more research is needed to fully understand the benefits of reflexology, it remains a popular holistic approach to enhancing health and wellbeing. As interest in alternative therapies grows, foot reflexology continues to be a helpful tool for improving general health, pain relief, and relaxation.

CHAPTER TWO

FOOT REFLEX ZONES

Understanding Reflex Zones in the Foot

The notion that various foot parts correspond to various body organs and systems forms the basis of foot reflexology. By mapping these reflex points, practitioners can apply precise pressure to target specific health issues. This section discusses in detail the primary reflex zones on the feet and how they relate to the overall functioning of the body.

Outlining the Reflex Points

Each of the foot's numerous significant reflex zones is linked to particular organs and body systems.

Below is a list of the main areas of focus:

1. Toes

- Reflex points include the head, neck, and brain.

Justification: The tips of the toes are connected to the brain and upper body. These points can be stimulated to treat sinus issues, improve mental clarity, and relieve headaches.

2. The foot's ball

Reflex points include the heart and lungs.

Rationale: The ball area symbolizes the heart and lungs. Here, applying pressure can improve cardiovascular health and respiratory function.

3. Foot Arch:

Reflex points are the digestive organs.

Justification: The arch area represents the digestive system, which includes the stomach, intestines, and liver. Stimulating this zone can help with digestion and relieve digestive disorders.

4. Heel

The sciatica and lower back are reflex points.

Justification: The heel area contains the sciatic nerve and lower back. Applying pressure to this area can help reduce lower back pain and sciatica.

5. The outer edge of the foot:

Reflex points on the spine.

Justification: The outer edge reflects the spine's alignment and health. Applying pressure to this region may improve posture and lessen stress.

6. The inner arch

- Reflex points include the kidneys and bladder.

Rationale: The inner arch is associated with the kidneys and bladder. Stimulation can help with detoxification and urinary health.

Reflexology's Impact on the Body

The body's response to reflexology is the result of intricate interactions between energetic and physiological processes.

The following impacts on general health may result from applying pressure to reflex points:

The Response of the Body

1. Initiation of the neurological system:

A relaxation reaction is triggered by reflexology's stimulation of the nervous system. When pressure is applied to nerve endings, signals are sent to the brain, releasing neurotransmitters that promote pain relief and relaxation.

2. Improved Blood Flow

Reflex points can be pressed to increase blood flow throughout the body. Improved circulation facilitates more efficient toxin removal and improved tissue oxygenation, both of which are advantageous for overall health.

3. Hormonal Balance: Reflexology can influence hormone levels by supporting the endocrine system. Numerous bodily functions, including mood, metabolism, and stress response, depend on this balance.

4. Pain Control:

Reflexology may activate the body's natural pain-relieving systems. Stimulating reflex points can result in the release of endorphins, which lessen pain and improve feelings of wellbeing.

Energy Pathways

In addition to its physiological benefits, reflexology is believed to have an impact on the body's energy pathways:

1. The energy flow

Reflexology is consistent with the concept of energy flow, which is comparable to qi in traditional Chinese medicine. Blockages in energy pathways can cause both physical and emotional distress. By stimulating reflex points, practitioners aim to restore balance and encourage the unrestricted flow of energy throughout the body.

2. Comprehensive Healing:

By recognizing the link between mental and physical health, reflexology promotes a holistic approach to health. By focusing on reflex zones, practitioners can ease emotional stress and increase mental clarity, which supports a complete healing process.

3. Stress Reduction:

The deep relaxation that reflexology offers can significantly reduce stress levels. Stress reduction can lead to a cascade of improved health outcomes, including enhanced emotional stability, immune system performance, and sleep quality.

In conclusion

Understanding foot reflex zones is essential for reflexology practitioners and clients. By allocating reflex points to specific organs and systems, practitioners can effectively treat medical conditions and provide a thorough healing experience. The body's response to reflexology through energy pathways and physiological changes suggests that it may be a helpful therapeutic modality. As interest in alternative therapies continues to grow, foot reflexology remains a practical and effective way to improve health and wellbeing.

CHAPTER THREE

TECHNIQUES AND PRESSURE POINTS

Foot reflexology is a sophisticated technique that applies pressure to specific foot reflex zones using a range of techniques. These methods can lower stress, promote relaxation, and improve general health. This section covers both basic foot reflexology techniques and more sophisticated methods that use tools to achieve better outcomes.

Basic Techniques for Foot Reflexology

1. Preparation:

Create a Calm Environment: Make sure the area is comfortable, quiet, and free of distractions. Apply essential oils, play calming music, or dim the lights to encourage relaxation.

Client Comfort: Ensure that the client has easy access to their feet and is seated comfortably in a chair or in a reclined position.

2. Warm up:

Gentle Strokes: Start with light strokes across the feet using your palms. This warms the room and promotes relaxation. Focus on the ankles and tops of the feet to prepare for deeper work.

3. The Method of Thumb-Walking:

During the execution, you apply pressure to the reflex points by "walking" your thumbs along the foot.

Methodological Techniques:

Place your thumbs at the base of your toes. Apply constant pressure as you move your thumbs down toward the heel. To ensure even coverage, use a mild rocking motion. Pay close attention to the tense areas as you repeat this movement several times.

4. The Finger Motions:

Pinching Technique: Use your fingers to pinch the reflex points.

Methodological Techniques:

Pinch the area between your thumb and index finger with steady pressure. After a few seconds of holding, slowly release. The arch and ball of the foot can benefit greatly from this.

5. Motions That Rotate:

Using Your Hands: Make tiny circles with your fingers or thumbs over the reflex points.

Methodological Techniques:

Find a reflex point, like the arch of the digestive organs. Apply pressure and rotate it for 10 to 15 seconds in a clockwise direction.

Switch to counter-clockwise rotation for 10 to 15 more seconds.

6. Compression Method:

Applying Pressure: Use your fingers or thumbs to firmly press on reflex points.

Methodological Techniques:

Select a reflex area, such as the heel, for lower back relief. For 10 to 15 seconds, apply pressure to the point. Release slowly and gently.

7. Finally, relax:

Ending the Session: Gently rub the client's entire foot to help them relax and become calm. Encourage the client to reflect by asking them to take a few deep breaths and think about how they are feeling after the session.

Advanced Reflexology Techniques

For practitioners who want to improve their practice, using tools can increase the effectiveness of traditional reflexology techniques.

Here are some advanced methods using a range of instruments:

1. Foot Rollers: Foot rollers are cylindrical devices that apply pressure and stimulate the entire foot.

Methodological Techniques:

Request that the client place their foot on the roller. As you focus on different reflex points, instruct them to roll their foot back and forth. This technique can give you a more complete massage and increase circulation.

2. Acupressure Instruments:

Overview: Acupressure mats or devices offer a unique experience by applying pressure to multiple points simultaneously, unlike manual techniques.

Methodological Techniques:

Have the client lie down or sit comfortably while you apply acupressure. To allow their body to acclimate to the pressure, instruct them to use the device for a few minutes. This method can be particularly useful for long-term maintenance between reflexology sessions.

3. Massage balls:

Usage: Specific reflex points can be targeted with precise pressure from tiny massage balls.

Methodological Techniques: Place a massage ball on the floor and ask the client to roll their foot over it. Encourage them to focus more on areas that are sensitive or feel tight. This self-administered approach empowers clients to take control of their own foot health.

4. Essential Oils:

Use: Essential oils can enhance the reflexology experience through aromatherapy.

Methodological Techniques: Essential oils, like lavender for relaxation and peppermint for energy, can be diluted with a carrier oil. Massage the mixture into your hands and then into your foot before starting any reflexology techniques. When combined, scent and touch can enhance therapeutic benefits and encourage more profound relaxation.

5. Hot Stone Reflexology:

Overview: Using heated stones can apply deep pressure and warmth to reflex points.

Methodological Techniques: To warm smooth stones, use hot water or a heating pad. As you gently massage the foot with the stones, pay attention to the reflex zones. This technique can aid in stress reduction and relaxation by utilizing the soothing heat of the stones.

6. Foot Baths:

Preparation: Taking a warm foot bath is an excellent way to prepare for reflexology.

Methodological Techniques: Soak the feet for 10 to 15 minutes in warm water containing essential oils or Epsom salts. This can relax muscles and increase circulation before employing reflexology techniques.

In conclusion

Foot reflexology provides a range of approaches that can enhance the overall experience and effectiveness of treatments, from basic methods to complex tools. Professionals can provide tailored sessions that promote holistic health and address the needs of each client by mastering these techniques. Using reflexology to promote balance, relaxation, and well-being is the ultimate goal, regardless of whether thumb-walking is done the traditional way or with modern tools.

CHAPTER FOUR

REFLEXOLOGY FOR COMMON SITUATIONS

In addition to being a therapeutic method designed to promote relaxation, foot reflexology is a comprehensive approach that can treat a variety of common illnesses. By concentrating on specific reflex points on the feet, practitioners can enhance digestive and circulatory health, as well as lessen stress, anxiety, and sleep disorders. This section looks at reflexology techniques that might be useful for these common issues.

Stress and Relaxation

Stress and anxiety are pervasive issues in modern life that often lead to a range of physical and mental health problems. Reflexology can be a helpful tactic for managing these issues by promoting relaxation and restoring balance.

1. Stress-Reduction Reflex Points:

• **Solar Plexus Reflex Point:** Located in the center of the foot, just under the ball, this point symbolizes the solar plexus, the center of the central nervous system of the body. Stimulating this area can help you achieve emotional balance and reduce anxiety. To work on this point, gently press in a circular motion with your thumb on each foot for two to three minutes.

• **Heart Reflex Point:** This point is essential for emotional well-being and is situated near the base of the left foot's toes. By applying pressure here, you can promote calmness and help ease tension. Maintain a steady, firm pressure while taking deep breaths, allowing your body to relax with each exhale.

2. Ways to Become Calm:

• **Thumb Walking Technique:** This technique uses your thumb to "walk" along the reflex points, applying continuous pressure. It can be particularly helpful in reducing stress. Look for any areas that feel tight or sore, as these could indicate a build-up of stress.

• **Deep Breathing Integration:** Include deep breathing exercises in reflexology sessions. As you engage your reflex points, take deep, slow breaths. Breathe deeply through your nose and exhale through your mouth, allowing your abdomen to rise. This method not only promotes relaxation but also helps the body release emotional tension that has been stored there.

3. Improving the Sleep Quality:

• For many people, anxiety and stress are the main causes of sleep disturbances. Reflexology can help the body prepare for a restful night's sleep by calming the nervous system. Focusing on the spine's reflex points, which are located along the inner arch of the foot, and the brain's reflex points, which are located at the tips of the toes, can help relax the body and mind.

• **Evening Reflexology Routine:** Develop the habit of spending 10 to 15 minutes each night performing reflexology on your feet. This could be interpreted by your body as a signal to wind down, which will help you transition into a sleep-friendly state.

Digestive and Circulatory Health

Reflexology is also beneficial for digestive and circulatory health. By stimulating specific reflex points, practitioners can enhance digestion, lessen bloating, and increase circulation throughout the body.

1. Reflex Points for Digestive Health:

• **Stomach Reflex Point:** Located in the center, just under the ball of the foot, this point symbolizes the stomach. Pressing and massaging this area gently can help reduce indigestion symptoms like bloating and discomfort. Spend 3 to 5 minutes concentrating on this point using small circular motions.

- **Gallbladder and Liver Reflex Points:** These reflex points, which are close to the right foot's arch, support detoxification and digestion. Stimulating these points can reduce post-meal nausea and discomfort and support liver function.

2. Techniques for Digestion Relief:

- **Kneading Technique:** Using your fingers, apply pressure in a rhythmic motion while kneading the reflex points in the stomach and liver. This method can enhance blood flow to these areas and promote digestive health by mimicking the effects of massage.

- **Hydration Awareness:** When doing reflexology, make sure to consume adequate water. Drink water before and after your session to help support the removal of toxins and support digestive function.

3. Reflex Points for Circulatory Health:

- **Heart Reflex Point (Revised):** As mentioned earlier, improving circulation and emotional health depend on the heart reflex point. Regular stimulation can enhance blood flow and cardiovascular health.

- **Ankle Reflex Points:** The reflex points near the ankles serve as a representation of the circulatory system. Gentle massage can help reduce swelling and cold feet, two symptoms of poor circulation. Use a firm grip and alternate between light pressure and deeper strokes to activate these points.

4. Everyday life reflexology:

- Consider incorporating brief reflexology sessions into your daily routine to support digestive and circulatory health. Concentrated foot reflexology for even 5 to 10 minutes can be helpful over time.

- **Self-Reflection and Observation:** Keep a journal in which you document your symptoms and progress. By monitoring the effects of reflexology techniques on your digestion, stress levels, and overall well-being, you can identify which ones work best for you.

In conclusion

Reflexology offers a thorough approach to treating common ailments like stress, anxiety, digestive issues, and poor circulation. By understanding the specific reflex points and techniques associated with these conditions, practitioners can tailor their sessions to meet the needs of each client. Whether your objective is to improve circulation and digestive health or to encourage relaxation, reflexology can make a significant contribution to your wellness routine. In the end, this will result in a better feeling of equilibrium and wellbeing in daily life.

CHAPTER FIVE

INTEGRATING REFLEXOLOGY INTO DAILY TASKS

Foot reflexology is a simple method that you can easily incorporate into your daily routine to promote relaxation, improve general well-being, and improve health. Whether your objective is to create a self-care routine at home or research the benefits of doing so, knowing how to appropriately combine reflexology with other therapeutic modalities can lead to significant improvements in your physical and mental well-being.

Self-Care Routine with Reflexology

Developing a self-care routine based on reflexology can be a fulfilling experience that allows you to take an active role in your relaxation and overall health.

Take these actions to start a productive reflexology practice at home:

1. Setting the Scene:

• **Create a Calm Environment:** Select a quiet, comfortable space in your home where you can perform reflexology undisturbed. Soft lighting, comfortable seating, and calming scents can enhance your experience. Consider using essential oils such as lavender or eucalyptus to promote relaxation.

• **Gather Your Tools:** Reflexology can be performed with just your thumbs and fingers, but it can be enhanced by using a few basic tools. Consider investing in a foot roller, reflexology chart, or massage ball to more effectively target specific points.

2. Making a Timetable:

• **Make Time for Reflexology:** Make an effort to perform reflexology at least twice or three times per week. Whether it's an evening routine to help you wind down or a morning routine to help you start your day with clarity, consistency is crucial. Setting a specific time helps you create a routine that becomes a part of your self-care routine.

- **Length of Session:** As you become more adept at the techniques, gradually increase the length of your sessions, starting with shorter ones that last 10 to 15 minutes. Focus on the primary reflex points that correspond to your current needs, whether they are stress relief, digestion, or relaxation.

3. Techniques for Practice:

- **Basic Reflexology Techniques:** Start by using your thumb to lightly trace the reflex points. Focus on areas that feel tight or tender and apply varying pressures according to your comfort level. Additionally, you can use kneading and circular motions to enhance the effects.

- **Breathing and Mindfulness:** Include breathing and mindfulness techniques in your reflexology practice. While working on your feet, take deep, slow breaths and pay attention to your breathing. This combination of physical contact and mental focus can enhance the entire experience and encourage greater relaxation.

4. Tracking Progress:

- Self-Assessment Journal: Record your feelings in a journal both before and after each session. Any changes in pain, stress, or overall health should be noted. This can help you understand how your body responds to different concentration points and which techniques work best for you.

- **Changing Your Practice:** Using your journal, adjust your routine in light of your observations. If certain reflex points consistently provide relief, think about using them more often in your sessions.

Combining Reflexology with Other Treatments

By carefully integrating reflexology with other therapeutic modalities, its advantages can be amplified. Reflexology can lead to a more holistic approach to well-being when combined with yoga, massage, and aromatherapy.

1. Reflexology and massage:

- **Complementary Techniques:** Reflexology is a useful adjunct to traditional massage therapy. Incorporating foot reflexology into a full-body massage can promote deeper relaxation and provide additional benefits to the body overall. While a massage therapist works on the upper body, reflexology can focus on the feet, ensuring a comprehensive treatment.

- **Better Circulation:** By relaxing muscles and boosting blood flow, massage therapy amplifies the advantages of reflexology. Combining these methods can improve blood flow and lower stress levels, both of which enhance overall health.

2. Reflexology and aromatherapy:

• **Scented Support:** Reflexology and aromatherapy work together to enhance emotional equilibrium and encourage rest. Use calming essential oils, such as lavender or chamomile, during reflexology sessions. After diluting the oils with a carrier oil, apply them to the feet while working on reflex points.

• **Creating a Sensory Experience:** Aromatherapy's capacity to produce a multisensory experience can promote deeper relaxation. If the relaxing scents aid in relaxation and stress relief, your reflexology practice will be even more effective.

3. Reflexology and Yoga:

• **Mind-Body Connection:** Both yoga and reflexology place a strong emphasis on the connection between the mind and body. Yoga can increase strength and flexibility, while reflexology works on specific pressure points to promote healing and relaxation. Combining these practices can help you feel more balanced and well overall.

• **Including Reflexology in Yoga:** After a yoga class, consider performing reflexology on your feet to maximize the benefits of your practice. Focus on the reflex points that correlate to any tense areas that may have developed during your yoga practice to help release tension and promote relaxation.

4. Creating an All-Inclusive Self-Care Program:

• **Weekly Wellness Rituals:** Plan yoga, massage, reflexology, and aromatherapy into your weekly routine. For example, you could schedule a foot reflexology session on Wednesdays, yoga on Mondays, and massages on Fridays. This holistic approach can help ensure a well-rounded self-care program that considers multiple aspects of health.

• **Listening to Your Body:** Pay attention to how your body responds to these combined exercises. Adjust the frequency and type of therapies to suit your unique needs and preferences in order to preserve the effectiveness and enjoyment of your self-care routine.

In conclusion

Reflexology can significantly improve your everyday routine in terms of relaxation, health maintenance, and overall well-being. By creating a self-care routine centered around reflexology and exploring its potential integration with other therapeutic approaches, you can create a holistic approach to health that considers both physical and emotional needs. Regardless of your objectives—stress reduction, improved digestion, or improved circulation—implementing these techniques can lead to a more contented and balanced life. As you establish your self-care practices, remember that reflexology and its auxiliary therapies require consistency and mindfulness to be fully effective.

THE END